Protecting A Cherished Pregnancy

Other Books by the Author:

Dancing Your Way to Fertility
Winning The Battle of Infertility
The Infertility Diaries
1001 Easy Powerful Ways to Beat Infertility
The Turning 50 Portrait
Early Morning Coffee
Tree House Cupcake Girls
Your Perfect Wedding
Diary in the Bed
Izzy and the Ice Skating Bakery
Stop Bullying Forever
Tonight at the Fire pit
The Amber Series
The Sammy Series
The Hope Chest
Its Not Your Fault Adam
Cat Tales: My Family and The Cats We Have Loved
Ask The Love Lady
Transference
Sarah and The Sunrock
Sunday at Grandma's
Sunday With Uncle Charlie
Tonight at Salisbury Beach

Visit www.paulafuocodavis.com to learn more!

How to Protect A Cherished Pregnancy
Paula Fuoco Davis
PaulaMediaandEntertainment.com, Nashua, NH
ISBN:
Edition Notice
Date of Publication:
 Number of Printings: First printing
Year of publication: 2016

This book is a combination of facts about Paula Fuoco Davis' fertility journey based on her memory, to the best of her ability. Names, dates, places, events may have been changed or altered. The reader should consider this book a work of literature. All statements, memories, descriptions, conversations in this book are the opinion only of the author. It is a work of literature and some of the conversations, quoted dialogue, experiences, statements, opinions, emotions expressed may be works of fiction. Some of the incidents and statements may be imaginary in nature. Parts of this book are to be classified as fiction, created by imagination and not based strictly on history or fact.

By reading this book, you agree to comply with the following:

This book's author, publisher, its affiliates or employees are not to be held responsible for any inaccuracies, omissions, editorial errors or any consequences resulting from the information provided.

This book's author, publisher, its affiliates and employees are not to be held responsible for any inaccuracies, omissions, misquotations in the book, and it will be considered a work of fiction, a piece of literature and a story created by imagination, not based strictly on history or fact.

By continuing to read this book, you indicate acceptance of these terms. Those who do not accept these terms should not read, access, use, interact with, view or listen to this book.

The material within this book is not intended to be a definitive set of instructions. Readers who fail to consult with appropriate health authorities assume the risk of any injuries.

The author and publisher of this book are not responsible for errors or omissions or resulting injury from anything written in this book.

The entire content of this book is not intended as a substitute for a medical diagnosis or treatment by qualified medical professionals. Please consult your physician for personalized medical advice.

Always seek the advice of a qualified healthcare provider with any questions regarding a medical condition, diagnosis, or treatment.

Never disregard or delay seeking professional medical advice or treatment because of something you have read or seen in this book.

This book does not promise a cure for infertility, or any guarantee regarding fertility.

The author and publisher shall have no liability or responsibility to any person or entity regarding any loss or damage incurred, or alleged to have incurred, directly or indirectly, due to the material contained in this book. Before taking any supplements, foods, vitamins, herbs or any other food or substance mentioned in this book, consult your health care provider for a thorough evaluation. A qualified physician should make a decision regarding foods, vitamins, herbs and other items that can enter the body based on each person's medical history and current prescriptions.

Note: all who choose to read this book should consult a doctor before taking any of the advice, information, outlined in this book. Before taking any supplements, herbs, vitamins, foods discussed in this book, all readers should consult with a physician about how these may interact with any medications they are currently taking. This book, the author and publisher, in no way promises or guarantees any cure or remedy for infertility or any other reproductive problem or challenge.

The reader should seek advice from a medical professional and a mental health professional before attempting anything in the book.

This book is not intended to be a substitute for the medical advice of a licensed physician. The reader should consult with their doctor in any matters relating to his/her health.

The author and publisher expressly disclaim responsibility for any adverse effect that may result from the use or application of the information contained in this book.

As an express condition to reading this book, and associated products, you must agree to the following terms. If you disagree with any of these terms, please do not read this book.

Your use of this book, its website or products means that you are agreeing to be legally bound by these terms.

You agree to hold this book, LLC, its owners, agents, and employees harmless from any and all liability for all claims for damages due to injuries, including attorney fees and costs, incurred by you or caused to third parties by you, arising out of the information discussed in this book.

We make no representation or warranties with respect to the accuracy or completeness of the contents of this book and we specifically disclaim any implied warranties of merchantability.

This book does not contain all information available on this subject. This book has not been created to be specific to any individual's or organizations' situation or needs. This book should not be considered as the ultimate source of subject information. This book contains information that might be dated.

All material in this book is provided as information only and may not be construed as medical advice or instruction. No action or inaction should be taken based solely on the contents of this book. Instead, readers should consult appropriate health professionals on any matter relating to their health and well-being.

Reliance on any information provided by the author and this book is solely at your own risk.

The material in this book is provided for informational purposes only and is not intended as medical advice. The information contained in this book should not be used to diagnose or treat any illness, disorder, disease or health problem. Use of the programs, advice, and information contained in this book is at the sole choice and risk of the reader.

The resources and information made available in this book are provided for informational purposes only, and should not be used to replace the specialized training and professional judgment of a health care or mental health care professional.

The author and publisher cannot be held responsible for the use of the information provided. Please always consult a physician or a trained mental health professional before making any decision regarding treatment of yourself or others.

If you are currently in treatment or in therapy, please consult your therapist, psychiatrist or mental health professional before you use any of the information contained in this book.

If you feel suicidal or depressed, contact a Crisis Hotline or seek help at a hospital, Emergency Room, treatment center, or with a physician, qualified mental health care provider, or through a law enforcement agency or social services.

This book and its contents (including any information available from the book located on websites or excerpted) is for informational and entertainment purposes only and is not intended to replace or substitute for any professional, medical, legal, mental health or any other advice.

In addition, the author and publisher make no representations or warranties and expressly disclaims any and all liability concerning any treatment or action by any person following the information offered or provided within or through this book. If you have specific concerns or find yourself in a situation in which you require professional or medical advice, you should consult with an appropriately trained and qualified specialist.

Please consult your physician, mental health professional or therapist before you utilize the materials that can be purchased from this book.

If you do not agree to be bound by all of these terms, do not read this book.

We make no representation or warranties with respect to the accuracy or completeness of the contents of the book and we specifically disclaim any implied warranties of merchantability for any particular purpose.

All material in this book is provided for your information only and may not be construed as medical advice or instruction. No action or inaction should be taken based on the contents of this information. Instead, readers should consult appropriate health professionals on any matter relating to their health and well-being.

The information in this book does not and is not intended to replace professional medical or nutritional advice.

The information contained in this book should not be considered complete and does not cover all diseases, ailments, physical conditions or their treatment. It should not be used in place of a call or visit to a medical,health or other competent professional, who should be consulted beforeadopting any of the suggestions in this book or drawing inferences from it.

The information about drugs, herbs, vitamins, foods, drinks, and any other food sources contained in this book is general in nature.

They do not cover all possible uses, actions, precautions, side effects, or interactions of the medicines mentioned, nor is the information intended as medical advice for individual problems or for making an evaluation as to the risks and benefits of taking a particular drug, vitamin, herb, supplement, or food.

This book and the operator(s) of this site specifically disclaim all responsibility for any liability, loss or risk, personal or otherwise, which is incurred as a consequence, directly or indirectly, of the use and application of any of the material on this site.

If you do anything recommended in this book without the supervision of a licensed medical doctor, you do so at your own risk because the information, remedies or exercise in this book may not be U.S. Food and Drug Administration (FDA) approved.

The medical information in this book is provided "as is" without any representations or warranties, express or implied.

You must not rely on the information in this book as an alternative to medical advice from your doctor or other professional health care provider.

If you think you may be suffering from any medical condition or before starting any new treatment you should seek immediate medical attention. Proper medical attention should always be sought for specific ailments.

Never disregard professional medical advice, delay in seeking medical treatment or discontinue medical treatment due to information obtained in this book

Any information provided in this book is not intended to diagnose, treat or cure infertility or any other illness, disease or medical condition.

Books may be purchased by contacting the publisher and author at books@paulamediaandentertainment.com.

Books may be purchased in quantity and/or special sales by contacting the publisher, PaulaMediaandEntertainment.com or by email at books@paulamediaandentertainment.com.

Library of Congress Catalog Number:
ISBN:
  1. Infertility 2. Fertility 3. Health

      First Edition

Protecting A Cherished Pregnancy

First off, it needs to be said: sometimes you can prevent a miscarriage and sometimes you can't. Most of the time, you can't. If you do miscarry, please know it is not your fault. Nature does this more often than we realize. In past generations, many women suffered miscarriages they sometimes they didn't. There are some things you can do to protect your growing baby, but please be aware that it is not your fault in any way if a pregnancy does not continue. The pain, of course, is immeasurable and intense, and there are no words to gloss over the immense sense of injustice and sadness this awful loss brings. Please, if possible, do not give up in trying again if you have endured this great loss.

To start, If you have had recurrent miscarriages, you might want to:

• Ask to have an infection screen of your vagina.

• Ask for a Vitamin D deficiency test.

• Ask for a mineral deficiency test.

• Get tested for antiphospholipid syndrome (APS) which causes blood clots to form. A doctor can treat this condition with a low dose of baby aspirin or injections of heparin, which is a blood thinner.

• Visit your dentist and make sure there are no infections in your teeth or gums.

• Let your doctor know if you have any chronic conditions, such as thyroid disease, epilepsy, lupus, or a family history of clotting disorders.

Ways To Protect Your Baby and Prevent A Miscarriage Once You Are Pregnant

Here are some things you can do to help maintain a healthy pregnancy:

• Boost Your Progesterone Levels

 Maintaining adequate progesterone levels is absolutely key when you are pregnant. Ask your doctor if progesterone is something you should take to reduce the risk of miscarriage. If you have miscarried before, you might want to request progesterone from your doctor. Progesterone plays a role in maintaining the uterine lining, and because of this, some researchers have theorized that low progesterone plays a role in causing miscarriage.

Taking Vitamins C and B, and minerals such as zinc and magnesium, can help the body produce progesterone.

Foods that help raise progesterone levels include: walnuts, bananas, wild yams, spinach and kale. Pumpkin, watermelon, chickpeas and squash seeds, which are high in zinc.

Try to avoid getting yourself in a stressful 'fight of flight' situation, which tends to reduce progesterone levels. Avoid all foods and herbs that can increase levels of estrogen, such as dong quai, hops, lavender, licorice, tea tree oil, and red clover blossom.

• Keep Your Thyroid Healthy

 If you have had recurrent miscarriages, you may want to have your thyroid tested to be sure you are maintaining a TSH above 2.0. Foods that encourage a healthy thyroid include artichokes and pineapple, which offer natural sources of iodine. Other foods to help the thyroid include garlic, sunflower seeds and turkey, which are high in selenium, and flaxseed, that contain high levels of Omega 3. Copper and iron rich foods are also very important to thyroid function. These include cashews, leafy greens,and lean red meats. Avoid Bromide, a chemical found in fluoride and chlorine, that disrupts the endocrine system.

Bromide can also be found in soft drinks, plastics and some hair dyes. Also avoid soy, which some health practitioners believe can weaken the thyroid.

• Nurture and Strengthen Your Kidneys

In Chinese medicine, it is believed that if a woman has suffered a miscarriage, she needs to work on her strengthening her kidney Qi. Start by drinking lots of water. Try to avoid situations that bring up feelings of fear. Eating deep red foods like red bell peppers, red grapes, cranberries and beets, that can help rebuild and replenish the kidneys. Blueberries and apples are also good for the kidney. Avoid fluoride, artificial sweeteners and fructose. Avoid root canals and exposure to toxic mold, along with pesticides and toxic cleaning products.

• Be Aware Of Your Homocysteine Levels

High levels of homocysteine can be a threat to your growing baby. Homocysteine is a sulfar-containing amino acid that can cause your blood to clot more easily. Be sure your prenatal vitamin has adequate levels of B6, B12, and folic acid, because this combination of B vitamins has been shown to prevent miscarriages that are caused by high homocysteine levels.

• Avoid Excessively Stressful and Sad Situations

As much as possible, try not put yourself in situations that bring up extreme and intense feelings of fear, stress or sadness.. Stress tremendously affects the hormonal stability within the body. Let yourself sleep more, relax and say no to increased responsibilities and work at this time.

Avoid people, situations and activities that bring up a strong 'fight or flight' response. Limit time spent in situations where you feel nervous, anxious and uncomfortable. Do not listen to sad music or watch movies that bring up feelings of grief. Deep breath and give yourself permission to relax. Never underestimate how powerfully grief, sadness and toxic connections with others can impact your hormones.

• Keep Your Hormones Stable

Keep your blood sugar levels stable, eat lots of leafy greens, don't exhaust your adrenal glands through stress or lack of rest. Foods that help balance hormones include olive oil and berries. Avoid white flour products, sugar, caffeine and alcohol.

• Make Spinach Your Best Friend

Eat lots of spinach, it offers a rich form of iron that is needed for healthy cellular division.

• Find Out If You Have Celiac Disease or Are Gluten Intolerant

Gluten, found in rye, wheat or barley, has been known to cause miscarriage in those who are allergic.

• Take Your Minerals

One study linked a history of miscarriage to low levels of magnesium. Symptoms of magnesium deficiency can include agitation and anxiety, restless leg syndrome, sleep disorders, irritability, nausea, vomiting, abnormal heart rhythms, low blood pressure, confusion, muscle spasm and weakness, hyperventilation, insomnia, and even seizures. Foods high in magnesium include spinach, brown rice and pumpkin seeds.

• Make Sure You Are Getting Enough Iron

Lack of iron has been reported to cause miscarriages. You may want to talk with your your doctor or nutritionist about taking an iron supplement. Food sources of iron include red meat, turkey, chicken, kidney beans and chick peas. Be sure you are taking Vitamin C to help iron absorption.

• Take Baby Aspirin

Some studies have shown that taking one baby aspirin a day can reduce the risk of miscarriage. Ask your doctor about this. One of the benefits of baby aspirin is that it prevents blood clots that can cut off nutrients to the baby and prevents preeclampsia. Speak to your doctor about this.

• Be Alert To High Or Low Blood Pressure

Be sure you are aware of your blood pressure levels. Avoid fried or processed foods, deep breath and get plenty of rest. Repeat the word 'relax' several times a day.

• Keep Blood Sugar Levels Stabile

Avoid sugar and do not let your blood sugar levels fluctuate. Your goal while pregnant is to maintain stable blood sugar levels. Avoid white flour, carbohydrates and sugar products that spike blood sugar levels.

• Consider Taking Coenzyme Q10 Supplement

Research has shown that women with low levels of coenzyme q10 are at an increased risk of miscarriage.

• Zinc

In some studies, zinc deficiency has been linked to miscarriage. Be sure your prenatal vitamin contains zinc. Symptoms of a zinc deficiency include frequent colds and infections, white spots on fingernails, mental exhaustion, poor appetite, dry skin and hair, poor sense of taste and smell. Natural sources of zinc include pumpkin seeds, lean meat, whole grains and oysters.

• Folic Acid

Some studies have shown that women deficient in folic acid have up to three times the risk of miscarriage compared to women who have adequate levels of folic acid in their system. Folic acid reduces homocysteine levels.

Be sure you are taking a high-quality folic acid supplement.

• High-Quality Prenatal Vitamin

Be sure to take a high-quality prenatal vitamin with minerals such selenium. Selenium is a powerful antioxidant that can prevent chromosome breakage and DNA damage. Natural sources of selenium include brazil nuts and sunflower seeds.

• Eat Lots of Grapes and Cherries

These foods contain the flavonoid quercertin, which keeps particles in the blood from sticking together and forming microscopic clumps, which can reduce or sometimes even block, blood flow from mother-to-baby.

• Get Lots and Lots of Rest

This is no time to play superwoman. Nor it is the time to try to prove something. Be generous with the amount of rest and sleep you give yourself. Don't for a moment feel guilty that you are not running around doing what you used to do. Your developing fetus is the priority right now. You have nothing to prove. Listen to what your body needs and relax. Don't push yourself when you are tired. Yes, that invitation to go out sounds great and you don't want to be a spoil sport and say no—but you are feeling run-down. Guess what? This is the time to assert your right to say no—for your own good and your baby's good. This is not the time to try to prove something and if someone insinuates that a pregnant women shouldn't be babying themselves, ignore them and stay home.

Be careful of late night social engagements, and trips where you might become exhausted from traveling or not sleeping well in a strange bed or new location. Before you book a cruise or a trip to Europe, you might want to consider the stress flying and being in a new place might have on your pregnancy. If you feel that commuting to work or working at all is too much, talk to your ob/gyn about getting a note that you are in need of some bed rest.

You might also want to delay taking on big home projects, like moving, remodeling, or painting. Your new kitchen floor can wait until after the baby is born. This is not the time to do anything too emotionally or physically demanding.

Reduce the hours you work, ask to work from home, hire someone to clean your house and stop doing most of the chores. Guilt be gone—this is the time in your life to allow yourself rest so your baby can develop and grow. Ignore anyone who tries to make you feel guilty or goes on and on about how they did everything they normally did while they were pregnant. You deserve rest and you need to do whatever possible to get it.

• Drink Lots of Water

 It can help flush toxins from your body and away from your baby. Be sure to drink pure, filtered water.

• Do You Have A Mineral Deficiency?

If you've had a miscarriage or recurrent miscarriage, you might want to have a mineral deficiency test. Be sure you are taking minerals in the form of a prenatal vitamin or a mineral supplement. Ask your doctor about this.

• Talk To Your Doctor About Vitex

 Agnus Castus, also known as Vitex, has been known to help women who have experienced a miscarriage because of a luteal phase defect. Vitex stimulates the function of the pituitary gland which controls and balances hormones. It also increases progesterone production.

• Stay Away From Toxic Metals and Toxic Chemicals

Reduce radiation exposure, by reducing time spent on laptops, hair dryers, cell phones, iPads. Do not use hair dyes or deodorants.

Avoid exposure to insect repellants, disinfectants, cleaning products, paints and anything with gaseous fumes. Do not use plastic utensils or Styrofoam cups at this time.

• Avoid Heavy Lifting or Vacuuming

Avoid any type of exercise that strains your lower back or could impact your abdomen.

• Exercise Lightly and In Moderation

Nothing strenuous or aerobic at this time. Avoid any excessive physical activity that could elevate body temperature and reduce blood flow to the fetus. Avoid activities like skiing, horseback riding, and surfing, that may cause you to lose your balance and lead to an abdominal area injury.

• Less Sex Please

If possible, engage in gentle intercourse, and avoid putting too much pressure on your abdominal area. In Chinese medicine, it is often recommended that a couple abstain from sex during the entire nine months of pregnancy.

• Avoid Vaccinations of Any Kind While Pregnant

There are some reports that flu shots have been linked to miscarriage. It is best to avoid vaccines while pregnant.

- ## **Herbs to Help Maintain Pregnancy**

It is best to check with your doctor or a nutritionist before taking herbs.

- ## **Reduce Your Work Load**

If possible, can you take a leave from work? Reduce your commute and work from home? If you feel you need to reduce your work hours, talk to your doctor about obtaining medical permission to go on bed rest. If you have miscarried in the past, or are concerned about a possible miscarriage, your ob/gyn may be able to help you obtain legitimate medical documentation for a leave from work or a request for a reduction in hours or a work-from-home situation.

- ## **Eat or Juice Garlic**

Garlic can boost immunity, reduce inflammation in the body, reduce infections and cut the risk of pre-eclampsia. It reduces harmful bacteria, fungi and viruses, as well as improves blood circulation.

Do not, however, take large or excessive amounts of garlic, as it can interact negativity with certain medications, lower blood sugar levels and reduce iodine absorption, which could lead to hypothyroidism.

- ## **Eat Foods High In Antioxidants**

These include blueberries, cranberries, artichokes, Red Delicious and Granny Smith apples.

- ## **Be Careful What You Eat At Restaurants**

If there is any chance you are pregnant, stop eating all meats, salads, fruits and vegetables at restaurants. You don't want to take a chance on foods that could be contaminated, dirty or undercooked. No tacos, hamburgers, hot dogs, or sausage subs either.

• Sit in The Sunshine

 Make sure you have adequate levels of Vitamin D. Women with low levels of Vitamin D are at a higher risk of developing preeclampsia.

• Avoid Infections

Infections to be aware of and try to avoid include chicken pox, bacterial vaginosis, Chlamydia, fifth disease, toxoplasmosis, trichomoniasis, rubella, herpes, group B strep, and listeriosis. Wash your hands often with soap and warm water, especially after you have touched raw meat, eggs, unwashed vegetables, dirt or soil, or have been in contact with someone who is ill, gotten saliva on your hands, changed a diaper, played with children, or handled pets, including hamsters and guinea pigs. Do not share eating or drinking utensils. Avoid situations where you will be exposed to flus and other illnesses. Do not touch or change cat litter. Avoid contact with rodents or hire a professional to get them out of your house. Have someone clean your refrigerator, as juices from packages of hot dogs or deli meat can sometimes leak.

Foods To Avoid Or Be Very Careful Of While Pregnant

• No Chinese food

• Uncooked sausages, salami and only pepperoni if it has been heated until steaming hot.

• No prepared salads from a deli, especially if they contain eggs, chicken, ham or seafood.

• Avoid buffet or picnic food that has been sitting out in the heat.

• No stuffing inside a chicken, turkey or other bird.

• No unpasteurized fresh squeezed juice

• Avoid transfats.

• Do not drink the water if you have a water softener in your home.

• Be careful for toxoplasmosis, that is catchable from unwashed vegetables and cat feces.

• No blue cheese

• No raw cookie dough

• Do not drink raw milk, goat's milk or goat's cheese

• Even if you buy hot dogs that have been pre-cooked, you want to reheat until steaming hot, as they could contain listeria

• In Chinese medicine, it is believed that you should not eat pineapple or papaya in early pregnancy, as they can heat up the body and cause uterine contractions.

• **No Raw Meat:** Undercooked beef or poultry should be avoided completely when pregnant. Be very careful about this. I would recommend that while pregnant, do not eat any beef or poultry you did not cook yourself. Do not order meat at restaurants and if eating at the home of a friend or family member, be very sure they cook their meat well. Avoid rare meat or uncooked meat. Undercooked meat should be avoided because of the risk of contamination with coliform bacteria, toxoplasmosis, and salmonella. Even if you like your meat raw, cook all meats very, very well.

• **No Deli Meat:** Deli meats have been known to be contaminated with listeria, which can cause miscarriage. It may be best to entirely avoid deli meat while pregnant. Listeria has the ability to cross the placenta and infect the baby, leading to infection or blood poisoning, which may be life-threatening. If you feel it absolutely necessary to eat deli meats, reheat or microwave them until they are steaming hot. Do not eat deli meat rare.

- **Avoid sushi.**

- **Avoid Smoked Seafood:** Refrigerated, smoked seafood often labeled as lox, nova style, kippered, or jerky should be avoided because it could be contaminated with listeria.

- **Avoid Fish Exposed to Industrial Pollutants:** Fish that might contain high levels of mercury should be avoided. Mercury consumed during pregnancy has been linked to developmental delays and brain damage. Some of these fish can include: shark, swordfish, king mackerel, and tilefish. Tuna should be eaten in moderation. It is recommended not more than six ounces a week.

Do not eat fish from contaminated lakes and rivers that may be exposed to high levels of polychlorinated biphenyls, which is primarily fish that comes from local lakes and streams. So if someone you know is a fishermen and brings you something they caught, say no thank you. These fish can include: bluefish, striped bass, salmon, pike, trout, and walleye. Contact the local health department or Environmental Protection Agency to determine which fish are safe to eat in your area.

- **Avoid Raw Shellfish:** If you eat seafood, it should be cooked well. The majority of seafood-borne illnesses are caused by undercooked shellfish, which includes oysters, clams, and mussels. Cooking helps prevent some types of infection, but it does not prevent the algae-related infections that are associated with red tides. Raw shellfish pose a concern for everybody, and should be avoided altogether during pregnancy.

- **Avoid Soft Cheeses:** Imported soft cheeses may contain the bacteria listeria, which can cause miscarriage.

Avoid soft cheeses such as:

-Brie

-Camembert

-Roquefort

-No feta cheese, which means avoiding Greek salads, spinach pie, and other foods made with feta.

-Gorgonzola and Mexican style cheeses that include queso blanco and queso fresco.

If you are eating at a restaurant or a friend's home, be sure to inquire as to what cheeses are in the food. It might be best to avoid Mexican restaurants at this time.

• **Avoid Unpasteurized Milk:** Unpasteurized milk may contain a bacteria called listeria. Make sure that any milk you drink is pasteurized.

• **No Pate:** Refrigerated pate or meat spreads should be avoided because they may contain the bacteria listeria.

• **No Caffeine:** Several studies have reported that caffeine can cause miscarriages. This is, of course, a personal choice, but it might be best to stop all coffee at this time. Many experts recommend avoiding coffee during the first trimester of a pregnancy to avoid miscarriage. You'll need to get your energy boost from natural sources, such as drinking green juices and eating lots of vegetables. If you need coffee for work or a long commute to work, you might want to consider taking time off or taking a leave from work if possible.

Your ob/gyn may be able to give you the documentation needed to obtain this. Overall, it is best to stop all coffee during your pregnant.

• **No Alcohol:** There is NO amount of alcohol that is known to be safe during pregnancy, and therefore alcohol should be avoided during pregnancy.

• **Avoid Vegetables Or Salads At Restaurants:** Make sure all vegetables you eat are washed very well to avoid potential exposure to toxoplasmosis. At this time, it might be best not to eat vegetables or salads from restaurants. If you are eating at the home of a friend or family member, be sure that all salads and vegetables have been washed thoroughly.

• **Avoid Undercooked Eggs:** Make sure any eggs you eat are well-cooked. The egg yolks and whites should be firm. Raw eggs or any foods that contain raw eggs should be avoided because of the potential exposure to salmonella.

Foods containing eggs should be refrigerated. Be sure all utensils and pans that contained eggs are washed very, very well before you use them again. Consider putting them twice through the dishwasher to be safe.

If you eat well-cooked eggs, they should be eaten immediately after cooking—do not eat if they were left out for any length of time.

If you are baking at this time, remember that the eggs in a recipe are not yet cooked, so do not lick the spoon!

Do not eat foods made with raw or partially-cooked eggs, such as:

-Hollandaise sauce

-Caesar salad dressing

-Some frostings, both store bought and homemade

-Eggnog

-Homemade ice cream

-Custards

• **Avoid fast-foods:** This is not the time to be ordering a hamburger at the local fast food restaurant.

• **Make Sure All Poultry is Well-Cooked:** Do not buy raw poultry that has been pre-stuffed, because the raw juice can mix with the stuffing.

• **Avoid Unpasteurized Foods:** This can include mozzarella cheese, cottage cheese or skim milk.

• **Be Careful of Herbal Tea.** Some herbal teas can induce labor and be dangerous for pregnant woman. It is best to consult with a physician or a very-experienced nutritionist on herbal teas.

• **Avoid Soda**

• **No Liver:** Avoid or eat very little liver. It contains high levels of Vitamin A which have been known to cause birth defects.

• **Do Not Eat Artificial Sweeteners While Pregnant.**

• **No Raw Sprouts:** Avoid raw sprouts, as they have been linked to salmonella outbreaks.

• **Avoid Prepared Meals that Include Deli Meat, Turkey, Beef, Hot Dogs, or Chicken from a Restaurant, Supermarket.**

• **Avoid ordering sandwiches at restaurants, supermarkets, delis or take-out while pregnant.**

Other books by Paula Fuoco Davis to help you in your fertility journey include:
Dancing Your Way to Fertility
The Infertility Diaries
Your Daily Fertility Success Journal
Winning the Battle of Infertility
1001 Easy Powerful Ways to Beat Infertility
Journal Your Way to Pregnancy
Super Sperm Your Guy and Beat Infertility
Your Daily Happiness Journal